1

My Personal Peripheral Neuropathy Story

Nerve Damage Symptoms
and Challenges By: Jim Lowrance

By: James M. Lowrance   © 2014

TABLE OF CONTENTS:

INTRODUCTION:

According to reputable medical sources, there are more than 100 identified types of Peripheral Neuropathies (PN) that are experienced by between 15 and 30 million people in the U.S. and at least 130 million people, globally (statistics vary somewhat among sources). While there is such a large number of PN types, all of these conditions boil down to one thing...nerve damage resulting in pain or failure of them to function properly. Nerves become changed with PN, in their reactions to pain and other physical sensations. This is due to either their sheaths (e.g., the medullary, myelin, or neurilemma) being damaged by diseases affecting them or from the nerves themselves being damaged or pinched/impinged; potentially affecting both large and small fiber types. The types of nerves themselves that can be affected, include "sensory" (sense of feel), "motor" (muscle strength-control) and "autonomic" (organ/glandular functions). Certainly in many cases, it is a combination of both large and small fiber nerves that are affected to varied degrees between each PN patent. In the more rare cases, temporary nerve damage can occur due to a viral infection that settles into certain nerves of the body.

This causes damage to them that is usually reversible, occurring in the myelin sheaths of the nerves (Chronic Inflammatory Demyelinating Polyneuropathy).

In this book, I will be sharing my own story regarding my experiences with PN, as a thyroid disease and diabetic patient; my also having experienced other negative metabolic manifestations. These include fatty liver disease and vitamin deficiencies, that were contributing factors in my case of nerve disease.

Heading 1:

Chronic Stress Plays a Role in the Development of PN

How do I know that the statement made by this chapter's heading is true? I not only know this because reputable medical websites state it to be so (those with MD backing) but also because I personally began to experience PN symptoms, years before I was diagnosed with diabetes or other major contributing diseases. I firmly believe stress to have been a major contributing factor in my own case of PN. Am I calling "chronic stress" a disease? No, I am not directly saying it is a disease, although it is very tempting to do so because of it's detrimental effects on the human body in so many ways. Medical sources have long known about the connection of highly experienced stressors, to the development of heart disease, bowel diseases, hypertension, sleep disorders...I could go on and on.

So, severe stress certainly plays a part, not only in the development of PN but also in the ongoing effect it has on a person who has developed it. In short, it can be a symptom aggravation factor, at the very least.

Chronic stress in my opinion, based on my many years of source-reading on the subject, can bring PN to the surface more quickly in people who are predisposed to developing it. This includes those with a family history of PN, diabetes and/or autoimmune diseases. It can also cause exacerbation periods of the disease in those who have already began to experience it; meaning times of significant symptom-worsening. Since a definitive cause for PN is not found in approximately 1/3 of people who develop it – which means it is "idiopathic" (unknown cause), could it also be true that chronic stress is a candidate for the cause in many of these idiopathic cases? Also, just so that it is not misunderstood, these unknown-cause cases of PN, present with actual nerve damage that can be seen with medical testing and they are not simply psychosomatic patients; meaning those with imagined nerve damage symptoms.

How was stress a factor in my somewhat slow developing case of PN? One major stressor I experienced beginning in approximately year 2002, was when I was fulfilling the duties of being a property manager.

I was performing maintenance, rent collection and gounds-keeping for a 100 unit mobile home park, containing mostly full-size trailer homes. I knew beyond doubt that the occupation would be very stressful, due to seeing the struggles experienced by the former Park Manager, who trained me for several months before I took on the job. It actually ended up being far more stressful than I had anticipated and I was only able to continue with the position for 2.5 years, in order to keep my sanity. I simply was not cut out for the job and apparently lacked the intestinal fortitude – as they say, to fulfill the occupation. I was actually offered ownership by the then-owner, who had contracted prostrate cancer and was actually dying from the disease but who didn't let anyone know this, beyond his closest family and friends. I declined ownership offers however, in spite of the significant profit the mobile home park was purportedly making; being a property with no liens/mortgages against it. The owner was in full possession but the retiring manager he had in place, who was at that time in his 70s, was needing to retire. Once he did retire, he passed away with 5 years of resigning his position with the mobile home park. In his case, chronic alcoholism contributed to his declining health and most likely, to the shortening of his life.

Coincidentally, the owner himself was also a chronic alcoholic, although the cancer was the most direct cause of his death.

The owner knew the resigning manager was not a good prospect to take over ownership, due to his age and his severely declining health, even if he became owner and placed a new manager in charge of the property. I was relieved with the realization that I did not opt for ownership, once I was in the property management position for a few months because it was possibly the most stressful and thankless job position I had ever undertaken. The greatest difficulty was not the gounds-keeping, landscaping and maintenance needs (I usually enjoyed those) but rather the dealing-with of extremely contrary people who rented spaces in the park for their trailer homes. Not only was collecting rent from some of them, harder than squeezing blood from a turnip but an unexpectedly high number of problems arose, due to some of them being neglectful and abusive to the park property.

Some tenants would not insulate their water pipes properly even with repeated warnings, so that freezing and breakage of them would not occur during wintertime.

While their own burst pipes was their problem, it would also cause a large loss of water from the water main, such as when pipes would burst over night and hundreds of gallons of water flowed from the main pipe, which had a meter on it and was paid for by the park (water and sewage was covered by tenant's rent fees). A tenant knowing their pipes were burst during the night, would often not even bother to call the emergency property maintenance phone number. Among other things, this number was provided to tenants for these type emergencies, such as contacting me to turn off the water main to repair broken water lines. After all (they must have thought), it wasn't their money being lost due to the massive water flow from a broken line, so they simply didn't call! But, if there was a problem with the park's water outlets, preventing them from having proper water pressure in their home, they would call immediately, even if it was 2:00AM in the morning! The amount of inconsideration by tenants was beyond what I could have ever imagined. I was one of those types of individuals, previous to my property management job, who saw everyone as being basically good people but this experience was a wake up call for me (literally and figuratively) and I realized how extremely selfish the basic nature of many people can be.

With that said, I still realize that there are many great, caring and basically good people in the world.

I noticed early into this 2 and ½ year experience, that I was having unusual nerve symptoms. I simply chalked this up to stress and tiredness for a time but with the frequency and intensity of my symptoms increasing more with passing months, I knew a negative change was occurring in my body. My symptoms included strange, neurological headaches that literally seemed to radiate ("referred pain") into other areas of my body. I also began to notice a strange tenderness on the top of my scalp, which I can only describe as being similar to the sensitivity one might have after receiving a sunburn on top of their head.

This is actually a symptom that is sometimes reported as being experienced by fibromyalgia patients but it is one that I continue to experience to this day, as part of my own PN condition (no two people are exactly the same). I also began to notice that my feet would burn and tingle at night after I retired to bed for a night's sleep; if I was allowed to get one!

Again, I simply attributed these symptoms to the stress of the property management job and I tried not to concern myself a great deal about it. I had more than enough on my plate to be concerned with already, without adding fears regarding my health to all of it, or at least I thought so at the time.

Heading 2:

When My Symptoms Finally "Hit the Fan" So-To-Speak

At one point early into my tenure as property manager for the 100 unit mobile home park - but long enough to already become totally stressed out, I was performing tree limb cutting and removal with my son helping me. I noticed while doing the strenuous work that my muscles seemed to fatigue very easily and that the headaches and scalp-sensitivity would occur more easily and with stronger effect, with each passing month.

At one point, I simply felt ill, as if I was experiencing a viral type illness. I developed hives on many areas of my body, which was a totally new symptom for me. I actually decided that I must have come into contact with a poisonous plant or one I was allergic too, while performing my gounds-keeping duties.

The problem was however, that this illness lingered for weeks, which included low-grade fevers, so with some prompting from my wife, I finally made a doctor appointment.

My doctor said that he felt I might be experiencing a food allergy and so he prescribed me an antihistamine and sent me home with the directions to observe what I was consuming in my diet and to eliminate any foods that I seemed to be having this reaction to. I attempted to do this but in the mean time, more symptoms began to manifest, including severe anxiety with panic attacks and night sweats. I would actually leave the outline of my body in sweat, on the bed I would be sleeping on and this was something I had never experienced before. I also noticed that the tingling I had experienced before, in my feet was now also occurring in my arms and hands, plus I continued to experience the easy fatiguing of my muscles, even with movement of them that was only moderately strenuous and sometimes even mildly strenuous. I knew beyond any doubt that these symptoms were not imagined/psychosomatic and not from stress or anxiety alone. My tingling and burning sensations also began to be accompanied by occasional stabbing pains.

I made another doctor visit and the fill-in doctor who was taking the place of my usual primary care physician, immediately diagnosed me with "Generalized Anxiety Disorder" alone.

She wrote me prescriptions for an anti-anxiety drug, an SSRI antidepressant and a beta-blocker (hypertensive medication), although my blood pressure was within only high normal limits at the office visit. I asked the doctor before I left her office, if she thought that some medical testing of some type might be in order, in light of my symptoms and she offhandedly responded saying "Well, we could have your head examined." Not realizing that she was offended that I, as a patient would make a suggestion, I responded asking if she was referring to an MRI scan. She continued her patronizing and insulting tone by saying "Yes, we could order you a brain MRI." I then asked what the cost for this would be because I was dead serious about finding the cause of my highly unusual symptoms. She then told me the cost would be about $2,000.00, which I would have to pay as an uninsured patient. Of course I had to decline but I wondered why simple blood testing was not suggested by her, which I could have easily paid for out-of-pocket.

I want readers to understand at this point of my relating this experience that I know for a fact that most doctors are good, compassionate people, who really do care about their patients.

Most also do not take out their personal venting-needs on patients, for problems within their own lives. We must all still beware however, that these types of doctors do exist. When we realize we are under the care of one, it is time to change doctors. I also recommend researching doctor's backgrounds, best possible to avoid care by a non-compassionate one, by talking to other patients who are attended by them if possible.

Checking into a doctor's background can also be done by researching their ratings online. This should be done at reputable physician reviews sites such as "HealthGrades.com", "RateMDs.com" and "Vitals.com", all of which are recommended by WebMD.com, as reliable rating sources.

Unfortunately, I was not savvy enough myself at the time, on how to locate good doctors or to properly research my symptoms online. As a result, I greatly increased my anxiety by producing more self-induced fear regarding my symptoms. Some websites I came across, related my symptoms to MS (Multiple Sclerosis) and others had me worrying about whether or not I might be developing a psychosis of some type (e.g., schizophrenia or bipolar disorder).

I feared that my peripheral neuropathy symptoms, which seemed to be occurring worse in my right leg, were the result of a dreaded disease such as "ALS" - Amyotrophic Lateral Sclerosis (as called "Lou Gehrig's Disease"). There are several terms for this phenomenon that comes from online search popularity. It is a self-induced anxiety disorder that causes this type of fear/phobia about one's health and that was actually studied at one point by Microsoft Corporation. It causes one to believe they have the most severe diagnoses from online search and these terms include: "Cyberchondria", "Surf Diagnosis" and "Availability Bias". So, as wonderful as online information can be (I personally thank God for it), web surfers must beware that they can cause an induced phobic state regarding their non-definitively diagnosed illnesses, by improperly using online search or by trying to obtain a diagnosis, exclusively online. You simply cannot arrive at a definitive diagnosis for any illness, without the proper investigation by a qualified, licensed medical doctor and without proper medical testing. Blood testing for example, will diagnose many illnesses, without further lab or imaging tests being needed, due to most diseases and illnesses being detectable within the blood.

If other tests are needed however, one should still not despair because doctors are usually highly qualified in knowing what further tests are needed or to what type specialists a patient might need referrals to.

Many times, symptoms of PN for example, will be diagnosed in regard to causative factors via blood tests, which can diagnose thyroid disease, diabetes and metabolic syndromes. This includes pre-diabetes, fatty liver and lipid or glucose imbalances of other types. Glucose and lipids are sterol-containing metabolites, which work together and should be within reasonable balance to avoid some metabolic illnesses. When they fall outside of normal values on either the high side, such as with "hyperglycemia" (elevated glucose – the most common indicator of diabetes) or on the low side, being "hypoglycemia" (insufficient glucose – which can indicate diabetes and other glucose-reactive conditions), this will be detected most often with blood testing alone. The same is true of other common diseases, such as those affecting the thyroid gland. In my case for example, the first disorder to be found with blood testing in year 2003, was autoimmune hypothyroidism.

It was more specifically an underactive thyroid, caused by "Hashimoto's thyroiditis" – the most common hypothyroid condition in industrialized countries of the world, including the USA.

At the time of my thyroid disease diagnosis, I was also found to be borderline diabetic, meaning I was on the verge of seeing elevated glucose levels that could indicate adult-onset "Type II" diabetes. Once my thyroid disease was treated however, my blood glucose levels became better balanced and my blood testing, done 2 to 3 times yearly to monitor my "thyroid hormone replacement therapy", showed my glucose to continue remaining within normal range. This would change for me however, slowly over time unfortunately and my blood glucose began an ongoing elevation toward diabetes.

Heading 3:

One Major Disease Diagnosed and Two More To Go!

My Hashimoto's disease, not only helped to explain my muscle weakness, the tingling in the limbs of my body and my anxiety spells, since the disease can first manifest with a spell of "hyperthyroidism" (over-active gland) but it also explained my general feeling of illness. It also helped to explain my sudden weight loss, followed by my slow but continued weight gain from progressive hypothyroidism, following its initial onset.

My doctors over the years, monitored my thyroid treatment and kept my hormones related to the gland within proper balance (e.g. "TSH", "T4" and "T3") but they also continued to monitor my blood glucose via "Hemoglobin A1c" tests, which average your blood sugar levels over 60 to 90 day periods. This major diabetes-detecting test, showed me to be within good normal values for years after my thyroid disease was found, which had apparently contributed to my earlier borderline diabetes finding.

At one point however, my metabolic panel, which usually includes electrolytes, lipids and liver-kidney tests, showed that my liver enzymes were beginning to elevate.

This is a common finding in people who are becoming or who have already become obese. Mine began to elevate even though I was only moderately overweight. It is a metabolic reaction by the liver, in which it begins to store too many fat cells, to the point at which normal liver cells begin to die and flood into the bloodstream. When these enzymes, the main ones tested being the "ALT" (Alanine Transaminase) and the "AST" (Aspartate Aminotransferase), are only mildly elevated, this is not of great concern to an investigating doctor because it usually indicates early "Non-Alcoholic Fatty Liver Disease" (NAFLD). Obviously the disease is of a different type in alcoholics who are found to have elevated liver enzyme levels in the blood. With common NAFLD, blood levels of ALT/AST may eventually become moderately or highly elevated. This can indicate that the fatty liver is in danger of evolving into a hepatitis type condition called "Non-Alcoholic Fatty Liver Steatohepatitis" (NASH).

With this latter condition, natural liver cells can die much faster because the liver has then become inflamed, which can also lead to cirrhosis of the organ (lesions/scarring that can spread). NASH can eventually lead to the need for liver transplant because the affected person's lifespan can be significantly shortened by the disease.

My own NAFLD, also referred to as "fatty liver steatosis", has not evolved into the more severe hepatitis condition. My blood values of ALT and AST however, have reached concerning, elevated levels -- at times being more than twice that of the highest normal values. So, my NAFDL was my second metabolic related health condition to be diagnosed in approximately year-2007 – the first being thyroid disease, diagnosed about 4 years earlier.

According to reputable medical sources, "Metabolic Syndromes"of any type can contribute-to or cause PN symptoms, even without diabetes being present. What conditions actually need to be present for a person to be considered as having a "metabolic Syndrome", which is more easily reversed than is diabetes?

Well, the Mayo Clinic states this about the condition: *"Metabolic syndrome is a cluster of conditions — increased blood pressure, a high blood sugar level, excess body fat around the waist and abnormal cholesterol levels — that occur together, increasing your risk of heart disease, stroke and diabetes."*

Now to my third diagnoses – the big one related to my own peripheral neuropathy. Yes, you probably guessed it, the disease was diabetes that evolved after I continued to gain weight and did not improve my diet nor did I get enough proper exercise. So, my thyroid disease was diagnosed in year-2003, my NAFLD/Metabolic Syndrome in year-2007 and my diabetes in year-2013. I knew I was to blame for the metabolic syndrome and fatty liver, which led to diabetes, and I wanted to kick myself for adding yet another major problem to my declining health. To top it all off, I also developed Adult Onset Asthma, which is not directly considered a metabolic related illness. This lung problem ended up actually being diagnosed as "Mild CODP" (Chronic Obstructive Pulmonary Disease); the non-smokers type, this year of 2014. Unfortunately, diabetes leaves the body with less healing abilities and as a result, it can contribute to accelerating any other diseases present within the body.

I will also mention that I was found to be deficient in vitamin D and E and insufficient (near deficiency) in vitamin B12, which are all now treated but the vitamin therapies may not have reversed all damage done to my nerves, during my deficiency years. Any one of these deficiencies alone can contribute-to or even cause PN conditions in some people who experience them. There are other nutritional deficiencies that can as well and blood testing is usually the method for detecting them.

Due to my having these manifestations of illness, including hypertension and chronic anxiety as well, I found that I was left with the choice of either applying for Social Security Disability benefits at age 50 (I'm now nearing my 52nd birthday, this late year 2014), which includes medical benefits or to risk dying at a much earlier age. I desire to grow old with my wife if at all possible and to see more future grandchildren by my son and daughter (I so far have one granddaughter by my son), among other things I look forward to with a longer life. My struggle to continue working increased over an 8-year period, until I came to the absolute realization that SSDI was the obvious answer and I was approved.

My COPD and diabetes diagnoses came approximately 2 years after the SSDI approval. As was with me, depression can also set in, when you have been a hard worker all of your life but you eventually find yourself at the point of being unable to accomplish the same level of physical or stressing activities, at a fairly young age. In addition to my hormone and vitamin imbalances being treated, I am also treated with medication to control my diabetic nerve pain. This is via "Gabapentin" (Major brand name: "Neurontin"), which is an anticonvulsant/analgesic drug, originally developed to control epileptic seizures but that has also been found to be effective in controlling pain from PN conditions. Another drug offered to help patients with nerve pain, includes the other major band name: "Lyrica" (Pregabalin). Other than my daily regimen of medications, hormones and vitamins, my additional treatment options are to eat healthier, lose weight and to exercise regularly. These additional options, should be absolute and resolute decisions by all PN patients, especially those with a diagnosis of diabetes but sadly, many patients fail at practicing healthy lifestyle practices. Statistics by the American Diabetes Association, state that *"two out of three people with diabetes die from heart disease or stroke"*.

CONCLUSION:

Peripheral Neuropathy disorders can occur as a direct or indirect result of not only diabetes but also of Metabolic Syndromes and any metabolic related health condition. This includes hypothyroid disease, which decreases weight loss abilities, even when well treated, as patients with the disease (myself included) will attest. Symptoms of PN can include burning, tingling, weakness and stabbing pains/sensations in the extremities and actually anywhere within the body. PN typically first affects the "small fiber nerves" that receive and transmit superficial feelings (e.g. pain, hot, cold and simple touch). Large fiber nerves can also become affected as well however, and these are those that lead directly into the spinal cord. When large fiber nerves are damaged or impinged (pinched), such as with sciatica neuropathy affecting the back and legs, the pain can become far more severe. If organs of the body become involved (autonomic neuropathy), a failure or change in function of them can occur as well, including heart, sweat gland and lung functions.

Like they always say "if I had it all to do over again", I would have tackled these issues with more fervor regarding proper diet and exercise.

As most of us also say "It is so very hard to do!" In reality we make it harder for ourselves because more attention to enjoyable, yet healthy foods and more enjoyable ways to exercise can be accomplished if we simply research those foods and find fun ways to exercise -- or at least somewhat enjoyable ways! The onset or the worsening of PN can be halted just by doing these two basic things, in order to keep excessive weight off and to strengthen the most important muscles and organs in our bodies.

{See my other books on the PN subject by title}:

"Peripheral Neuropathy Causes and Treatments" (Published Year-2011)

"The Strange Symptoms and Challenges of Peripheral Neuropathy" (Published Year-2013)

(END)

Approximately 4,320 Words